I survived Ebola virus

A story of survival during pandemic times
Based upon Angeline Teah's story

Printed by Amazon.com, Inc., in the United States of America
ISBN: 9798634017136

First printing 2020.

Published by:
Palava Hut Publishing

I

My name is Angeline Teah. I want to share a personal story that began in late July 2014. During that time, I was living in New Kru Town with my three children, my father, my brothers and sisters, plus other relatives. I wouldn't consider ourselves as rich people, but we were definitely a very happy and traditional Liberian family. I was not employed back then. I operated as merchant and trader, by purchasing good items at low prices and selling them at higher price. This practice provided some profit and helped me sustain my children.

As I was living a regular life, I was unaware of the latent virus cases that began to increase in our city and in our country. I became conscious of the virus when one night my family was reunited at home and my father spoke about it. "Have you heard about a virus that is in our town and country?" he asked. I began feeling anxious and alarmed as my father was talking about it. He was advising me and my sisters to remain alert and take care of ourselves. He was talking with an eerie and fearful voice, "This virus is called 'Ebola' and people are dying from it." To which I asked, "Oh really? What do you mean by Ebola? What kind of virus is it?" "People are dying. You guys need to be careful with this deadly virus."

He further described the effects of the virus for us. He explained, "This virus goes through multiple stages while developing inside the body. Most of the patients realize they are infected once it's too late." My father told the history of the illness. Apparently, this was a virus that had existed for centuries but there hadn't been cases in a long time. He advised that we needed to take very good care of ourselves, emphasizing the special precautions needed when we were with other people.

My only thought at that moment was how could we prevent it and what were the necessary precautions. At the same time, I was very concerned thinking, what could we do to avoid getting infected from the virus in our daily life? That night I was unable to shake the news of this strange illness out of my head. Even though this was not a new virus, the information and the outbreak were new to me. It was the return of an old illness that remained dormant in our town.

The next day I visited the nearest grocery store to buy some items and food. A couple of weeks ago, everything seemed normal, and people were going through their daily lives. This time, it was astonishing to notice everyone else's awareness of the virus. Small groups of people and some others on their phones were talking about Ebola. I walked by a group of three people who were chatting with each other and I overheard: "We need to be careful, I heard people are dying from Ebola." I couldn't believe what I was hearing so I decided to step closer and join their conversation. "What is this disease you are talking about?". A lady answered: "It is a nightmare. People are getting sick from Ebola virus, but this is not a new disease. I remember stories about a lot of people dying from Ebola virus centuries ago. We thought it was eradicated, but it came back."

A man that was walking by, joined our conversation as

well. "I remember this disease existed many years ago. People would bleed from their nose, eyes, and mouth after getting infected by the virus." We exchanged nervous and anxious looks as he continued to explain. "The skin breaks out and rashes appear. Another symptom is diarrhea and in extreme cases people can die of dehydration." We were speechless, and he said before leaving: "Now that we know the virus is back, we must be extremely cautious."

One lady said, "The fact that we cannot see it until it is too late, makes it absolutely dangerous. People don't know they were in contact with the virus, until the symptoms become noticeable. They could be carrying and spreading the virus for days without manifesting any symptom." As I was leaving the grocery store, I tried to make sense of everything I had just heard. I felt my mind and body were on edge at that moment and I tried my best to remain calm, but there was a deadly threat developing around us already. It's hard to explain the feeling that invaded me.

As soon as I got home, I approached my father. "Hey Papay... It's true. People were talking about it in the parking lot, in the grocery store. Everywhere... I'm scared of everything I heard. The gruesome symptoms and how many people are dying. Is it really an invisible menace?" He responded, "I'm relieved that you believe me now and that more people are aware of it." He looked at me and said in a serious tone, "It is really dangerous and that's why I told you to take care of yourselves. I plead to you and your sisters to protect each other."

He called my sisters and we gathered around him. "I

know you are full-grown women and you have to provide for your families, but please be cautious. Protect yourselves and your children." My father did not know the precautionary measures, but he insisted to be careful.

II

I can tell you how the virus entered our family. My oldest brother, Bati, was a senior-level nurse. In our community, he was considered at the same level as a doctor. But I am unsure whether he was an official medical doctor or not. His wife worked as a nurse as well, but she was not on the same level yet.

Her uncle was infected by the virus at some point and he was abandoned by everyone later. All of us were aware of the potential threat and exposure, yet she couldn't abandon her uncle to his own misfortune. Secretly, she began visiting her uncle and taking care of him. My brother Bati was unaware of her actions. She didn't tell him because she knew that he wouldn't allow her to continue looking after her uncle. While taking care of her uncle, she failed to take precautionary measures. Even though she was a nurse, there was not enough information on how to prevent catching the virus. Her routine consisted of taking care of her uncle and then going to the hospital to perform her daily duties as a nurse.

One day while Bati was at work, his sister in law arrived at the hospital and looked for him. She explained in an anxious state, "Your wife is not feeling well. We just talked, and she is ill at home. She cannot move because she is very weak, and coughing a lot."

"Wait, what? She was OK when I left earlier." He was definitely shocked because he was aware of Ebola symptoms. "What are you talking about? I saw her this morning and she was alright. How is it possible?"

She answered, "I better be honest with you. She has been treating our uncle, but she didn't want to tell you. Our uncle was infected by the Ebola virus… I suspect she caught Ebola disease when she was treating our uncle." My brother was astonished, and it took him a minute to wrap his head around it. After a moment he was only able to ask himself, "How could she hide such a thing from me?"

My brother was hoping and praying that she had only caught a fever or the flu. But by the following day, her condition had worsened. Her eyes looked different, and she was coughing up small amounts of blood. Considering the symptoms, it was clear that she had caught Ebola and that he had been exposed to the virus as well. Nonetheless, he remained hopeful that she was going to get better eventually, so he decided to take care of her. He went to our father seeking advice. "Papay, I need your help. I think my wife caught Ebola when she took care of her uncle."

Our father was very concerned, but he agreed to help Bati and went to visit my sister-in-law. My brother and father thought that there was a possibility to nurse her back to health. It was at that moment that my father came across the Ebola virus.

A couple of days later, we received the sad news that her uncle passed away. The funeral was a very hard moment for us. It was a dark and rainy afternoon in which Ebola took the first victim in our family. We said our goodbyes as the casket was lowered to the grave. From a distance, I noticed my sister-in-law, she was trying to hold herself and look normal, but her facial expression looked totally deteriorated. She looked sick and weak. Her skin used to be lighter and fairer than ours, but her tone had darkened. I remember thinking: "Her uncle was an old man and he couldn't fight Ebola off. She's young and strong. She will get better soon." How mistaken I was.

Her condition kept decaying with every day that passed. At some point she was so weak, that she was unable to move her arms and legs. Since she wasn't getting any better, Bati and father decided to take her to the hospital. Unfortunately, the hospital administration refused to take her in. They explained, "We cannot take this woman, we won't be able to treat her." Therefore, they were forced to take her back home. Sadly, my sister-in-law died the following morning. After she passed away, it was evident that my brother wasn't feeling good either. He was sad indeed, but he looked weak and ill.

Around a week later, my father began wondering if we had seen or talked to Bati. We had given him some time and space, so he could mourn his departed wife. But when we arrived at his house, nobody answered the door. My father was worried, so we asked around with the neighbors. Perhaps someone could tell us where he was last seen or if anyone had been in contact. A neighbor told us, "Bati wasn't feeling well. He was last seen with the community pastor. I suggest you go to the church and ask around."

We went to the church and the pastor told us that my brother was there. We felt relieved until he said: "Bati was ill when he arrived. He was abstaining from food because he had been vomiting, but we have him eating again." My father was very upset at the fact that the pastor didn't contact us about my brother's condition. Once we saw him, we recognized the symptoms he was going through. It was indeed Ebola virus.

My father and I decided it was best to take Bati back home, he would be safer, and father could look after him. We noticed that my father didn't want to share too much information with us. Everytime we asked about Bati's condition, he'd respond, "He is doing well. You don't need to worry about him." We believed his words, we were happy thinking that my brother was getting better. But as the days went by, we saw my brother's condition deteriorating slowly. He was unable to hide the reality from us when my older sister paid them a visit. Bati's condition was critical, so my sister suggested we seek medical attention.

We took him to ELWA Hospital, where we found ourselves surrounded with other sick people. The hospital administration explained that they had run out of beds, and they were overwhelmed with the continuously increasing cases of Ebola. Since we didn't own a car, we couldn't risk carrying my brother back and losing our place in the line. We decided that we were going to stay overnight, considering the possibility that one patient could be discharged and a bed becoming available. That night my brothers, my sister, my father and I, slept outside on the hospital ground. The following day, there was an available bed for my brother and we left him in the hospital. We trusted that the nurses were going to take good care of him and we would later come back to a healthier Bati.

Later, my sister and I went to check on him, we wanted to make sure he was in a cleaner environment. We were petrified with the gruesome unveiling. The hospital must have been understaffed and the patients with Ebola were coming nonstop. You could feel death in the environment. There were kids and adults that had vomited and defecated themselves, the place reeked of urine and feces. There were flies all over the place. We could tell a lot just by looking at the sick people's eyes. You could see they were slowly running out of life.

"I can't stay here anymore. I have to leave now." I told my sister. Even though our brother was there, it was a very crude scene to watch. We really thought the hospital was the best place for him to get better. We thought we were leaving him in good hands with experienced nurses. Instead, we found ourselves witnessing a living hell and we couldn't bear to watch it.

The next day, my sister went to visit Bati. When she came back she told us, "He is doing well. His health is improving." We felt relieved that we were finally receiving good news. But my sister's expression was telling us a different story, she remained distant and quiet. "How is he improving? Considering everything we saw yesterday, I find that hard to believe." I wondered, but I wanted to believe in my sister's words and the power of God. We tried to make my sister join our conversation, but her response was: "I need to be by myself now."

My father could sense something was off, he went to the hospital because he wanted to see an improved Bati with his own eyes. We followed along to see my brother and speak to the hospital staff. A nurse gave us a devastating message. "I'm very sorry, but your son died last night. A lady came late last night and we gave her the news. She said she was the sister of the departed, and we assume she would give you the news." The information hit us like a ton of bricks. We arrived with the high hopes that my brother was healing, but he was already dead. "My son is gone! My son is gone!" my father lamented. He dropped hard on the floor and began slamming his back against the wall. We cried together.

III

A couple of days went by and our atmosphere was filled with sorrow as we mourned our departed ones. Our neighbors and other people from the community visited us in this hard moment. They came to pay respects to Bati and express their support during the funeral. Everyone knew that Bati and his wife had died from Ebola, along with her uncle. Therefore during these visits, it was evident that most people were afraid of getting too close to us. People were rejecting the food we were offering, they refused to take a seat at our table, and acted strangely towards us in general. I couldn't blame them, if it had happened to a different family, maybe I would be afraid to catch the same deadly virus. We simply appreciated their support and company.

My father was an older man, he already had a heart condition and a weak liver as a result of drinking alcohol. But after all this, his condition decayed. He began to show different symptoms than his usual ailments. We suspected he contracted Ebola from the days he assisted Bati. Father told us that he bathed him a couple of times, he must have come in contact with the body fluids and he didn't take precautionary measures. Or maybe he was feeling weak because of his current condition and the losses we went through.

During the following days, we took him to different hospitals and the doctors gave us different medicines, but he didn't seem to get any better. The doctors asked about his medical history, and we explained his current condition of heart and liver disease. They gave him different treatments, but nothing seemed to work. Even though my father was separated, our stepmother came to help us take care of him during this time of need. One of my sisters and I became suspicious about the possibility that he caught the Ebola virus, especially because we were following the medical instructions and he kept worsening. We confronted him and he couldn't hold it any longer. He broke down and apologized: "I am very sorry girls! I think I caught Ebola from Bati, but I was trying to hold it. I was in denial, but now I think I exposed you to Ebola too." We felt agitated and confused. "Papay! Why didn't you tell us this before?!" He explained that he was afraid we would abandon him and he was hoping he hadn't caught the virus. He apologized for exposing us, but he didn't know what else to do. Our father was consumed with guilt after the confrontation, or maybe the disease affected his mental state, but he was definitely acting different.

The house we lived in had one outdoor bathroom and one inside bathroom. Even though my father had always used the bathroom inside the house, he was now refusing to use it or bathe in it. Now that we were taking him to the outside bathroom, people in our community began observing and monitoring my father's condition. They asked us, "What's going on with your father? Where is he now?" By this time, the community was suspicious about my father's situation. A meeting was held by the community leaders, it was decided that the best option would be to transfer him to a hospital. Fody was an ambulance driver in the community, he had agreed to transport my father to the hospital. We felt dispirited as the days passed and Fody didn't show up at our house. We tried to contact him and ask other people to pass the message, but he never came. A couple of days later, we decided to take our father to the hospital ourselves. We couldn't carry him because he was too weak, so we went and looked for a taxi. Unfortunately, our father died on the way before we reached the hospital. It was a heartbreaking moment to see another family member dying as a result of the Ebola virus.

My father's death was very hard for our family. I remember one night we were praying together and he told us, "I'm going to be the last one that dies from Ebola in this family. You need to do everything you can to survive. Don't let Ebola take another member of this family." After his death, I had a conversation with my sisters. "This is serious. We must do something to save our family."

The entire community had isolated us and people began mistreating us. Our family was forced to 21 days quarantine. We couldn't go to buy groceries because we were not welcome at the stores. A storekeeper yelled at us, "Don't come here!! We don't want you in our store!!" They were afraid other customers would stop buying, if they saw us there. The family kids were forbidden to play with other kids or even go near other yards. One time our neighbor was yelling at me, "Do not let your children near our yard! We don't need to catch your family's disease!" I furiously yelled back, "You act as if my kids were defecating all over your yard!" We had a community water reservoir that was used to collect water, we were forbidden to go near it as well. We were mourning our departed loved ones, while the whole community treated us as outcasts. It was a very frustrating and demoralizing time of our lives.

One day, my older sister Teta and my stepmother began feeling ill. The symptoms they were showing were the same ones we had seen with my brother, my sister-in-law and my father. We were absolutely sure that they had caught the Ebola virus while taking care of my father. Our stepmother's sickness progressed rapidly. She was unable to eat anything, which caused her body to feel very weak and was coughing up blood. First we didn't have the numbers to contact the Ebola ambulance to transport her to the hospital, but we were able to get it later. When we contacted the number, the official told us they will be picking her up the following day. But they didn't show up. We contacted them again and they made the same commitment only to leave us waiting in vain. We couldn't wait any longer, her body was decaying faster every day. We contacted a taxi to drive us to the hospital, but my stepmother died on the way. When we arrived at the hospital, the nurses took her body and they refused to give it back. We couldn't even give her a proper burial, her body was taken to a mass grave by the government. We were taking one loss after another.

We were feeling isolated, not only because the community had us in lockdown, but also because the only communication device was taken from us. We owned a cellphone that we used for emergencies, to call an ambulance or taxi, but it was taken from us when our stepmother died. Since the hospital administration was trying to contain the virus, they didn't let us take any of her belongings and the cellphone was along the things they took from us.

The people in the community knew that our father was the food and money provider in our family. After a couple of weeks we were struggling tremendously. We were running out of food and other basic supplies to live. Our neighbors and other community members gathered together to consider my family's situation. It was decided they weren't going to sit back and let our family perish from the Ebola virus. Even though we were still under quarantine and treated like outcasts, our neighbors had good gestures with us. We were very thankful for their acts of kindness. For example, we were forbidden from going near the water reservoir or the stores, but they would bring water and food for us. They would leave the provisions out in the yard, since they were afraid to come in close contact with us. Unfortunately, not all days were so prosperous. We understood that the community had to look out for their own families as well, and they couldn't bring water and food every day. For this reason, there were some days in which we were unable to eat or drink anything. Our neighbors' good will helped us survive those hard days.

Somehow, our story reached the ears of the workers in a Non-governmental Organization (NGO). A female representative came to visit us one day, she wanted to know how we were doing and enduring the situation. "We are doing well in terms of eating, drinking and bathing. Our community has forbidden us from leaving the house, but they have been helping us. They bring us food and water. But when they can't bring us anything, we have to wait and hope they can afford to bring us something the following day." Before leaving, she agreed to bring us some food and water in the following days.

Teta wasn't getting any better, and on top of it all, I began feeling weak and sick as well. I remained hopeful that I hadn't caught the virus, I thought that maybe I was just tired and under a lot of stress. But then I started getting chills and shivers. One day I started coughing hard and noticed I was coughing up blood. I went and told my sister "I am coughing up blood Teta, I think I have the virus too." We saw each other with a very demoralized look. That moment we had to make a decision. So far none of our relatives that caught Ebola had survived. This virus seemed eager to consume our whole family, but we couldn't let the virus spread among our children.

We decided it was better to isolate ourselves in the living room. We demanded they stay away from the living room and not come any close to us. We would have preferred to quarantine ourselves in a clinic, but we didn't have a phone to call an ambulance. Staying in the living room was the best option we could think of. Some days after we had isolated ourselves, our younger brother joined us. He began showing symptoms of Ebola and he didn't want to expose the rest of the family to the virus.

IV

Our community decided to help us again, a neighbor drove my sister, my brother and me to the clinic. As we were arriving at Redemption Hospital, from a distance I recognized my children's father was outside as well. When I was getting out of the car, he approached me and said, "Angeline! Are you ok? What are you doing here?" He noticed my brother and sister were in the car as well, and I didn't have to answer, he already knew we were sick. "I am going to be here for a while. If you need anything, don't hesitate to ask for my help, ok?" To which I agreed, but I kept wondering what he was doing here to begin with.

The clinic was packed. Teta and I were in closer beds, but my brother was placed near the bathroom door. Since the clinic was so crowded and the bathroom was constantly being used, he was surrounded by a very unhygienic and dirty atmosphere. He hoped things would get better, but more people kept coming to the clinic. One hot afternoon he took his shirt off to take a nap. Someone took his shirt and cleaned themself after defecating. After this very disgusting experience, he decided he wasn't going to take it anymore. He slipped out of the clinic at night and tried to go back to the community, but was caught by the security members. When they questioned his reason for leaving, he said, "Nobody can heal in this filthy condition. This place is inhumane." Yet he was forced to go back to the same bed.

A few days later, the clinic decided it was best to transfer the Ebola patients to a larger hospital. The patient overflow caused unsanitary conditions. Teta and I heard that Ebola patients' names were being called to be transported to the larger hospital, we speculated of the possibility we might have been skipped. My sister panicked and said, "Are they going in alphabetical order? They're not even looking at us! I do not think they are going to call our names." I responded "I don't know, let's wait and see." Suddenly a nurse approached us and said "Both of you ladies will ride along with me to the other hospital." I responded, "Our brother is in this clinic as well, can he ride along?" The nurse responded "No, we do not have enough room. He will be transported on the next trip, everyone will be relocated to ELWA 3 Ebola Management Center." I thanked the nurse and waved at my brother as we entered the car.

Upon arrival, each one was given a bucket of water to clean ourselves. The refreshing gesture was welcomed and appreciated by my sister and I. This was a massive improvement from the horrible conditions we've previously experienced at the clinic. A bathroom became available and I was first to take a shower. As I poured the water over my head, I immediately felt a burning sensation in my eyes which I recognized as the smell and presence of chlorine in the water. I desperately exited the bathroom requesting a non chlorine-laced water to wash my eyes and face. I fussed at the nurse for not disclosing the bath water was laced with chlorine. The nurse apologized and responded that the chlorine was included in the water to kill the virus.

I warned Teta of the water as it was her turn to take a shower. I suspect she might have underestimated the level of chlorine in the water because minutes later she screamed out from the bathroom "My eyes are burning! I have chlorine in my eyes!" I shouted back at her, "I told you to be careful! I have to find the nurse, I'll be right back." The nurse and I return with a bottle of water to wash the chlorine out of my sister's eyes. When we returned, my sister was lying in front of the bathroom door and holding her leg. We rushed to her aid and I asked, "What happened?!" She responded, "My eyes were burning pretty badly and I couldn't wait any longer, so I decided to find something to wipe the chlorine from my eyes. I was unable to see clearly, I slipped and injured my leg." I expressed my unhappiness to the nurse and blamed her for our misfortunes. She repeatedly apologized. My sister and I were separated shortly after our baths.

I kept in contact with my children's father and I informed him that we were transferred to the Ebola Management Center. Every so often he would bring fruits and different food, which allowed me to eat a little better than the rest of the patients. However, my condition worsened shortly after our arrival to the new hospital. I became extremely tired and sometimes delusional. I was also very weak and incoherent. My body mechanics took more time and energy to work in accordance. I lost track of the days and struggled to stay awake.

I remember being awakened by a nurse to eat a little and take my medicine. I then recalled I arrived alongside my sister expecting my brother to join us. I mumbled to myself, "My brother and sister should be here with me. Where are they?" I gathered the energy to leave my bed and walked to the hospital's front desk to inquire about my brother and sister. The lady at the front desk wasn't giving me a straight answer, she told the guard to radio the supervisor to come to the front desk. I grew frustrated with the front desk person and noticed a younger lady that arrived the same time as Teta and I. I then approached her and asked "Hey, remember I arrived here along with my sister? Have you seen her?" The young lady responded by saying "Your sister died." I responded "What!? Are you telling me my sister died?" She responded, "Yes, your sister is dead." and walked away heartlessly. I was shocked and frozen. I had questions like "When, how and why?" I suddenly felt lonely thinking to myself "My sister, my best friend is gone". I had slowly become conscious that my family was losing the fight against Ebola virus.

I've lost Bati, his wife, my father, my stepmother and now my sister Teta. Was it only a matter of time before I perished as well? Then a thought hit me, "Where is my younger brother? I need to find my brother." I tried to walk but I instantly felt lightheaded and lost my equilibrium, then everything went black.

I woke up laying in bed and thought of my sister and family. I was overwhelmed by questions like, "Why am I fighting to live? Will I survive this battle? Why is this happening to me? Is today my last day?" My thoughts were interrupted by a nurse walking over to my bed and saying "Are you awake? Your brother keeps requesting to see you. We told him you were asleep but I don't think he believed us. Would you like to get up and be with your brother? " Of Course I wanted to be with my brother. At this point he was my only support system at the hospital. The nurse assisted me in sitting up and walking over to my brother's bed. As we approached my brother I noticed him fussing with his caretaker and refusing to take his medicine. He uttered "No! Where is my sister?! Don't touch me! Where is my sister?!" We got closer to his bed and I said "I am right here, I am here with you" as I touched his hand. He turned, recognized me and smiled. He then said "They said you were asleep but I didn't believe them. I am so happy to see you. How is everyone? Where is Teta?" I slowly sat down in a chair next to his bed, held his hand and delivered the news that Teta, our older sister, was dead. He squeezed my hand and we both cried together. We chatted, remembered and laughed at the many silly antics we witnessed growing up with our sister Teta. It was refreshing trading childhood stories with my brother. A moment later I grew fatigued and decided to return to my bed. My brother and I vowed to survive and beat the virus.

I was awakened by the coughing sounds of several patients in the beds near me. I opened my eyes and noticed a room filled with very ill people. I thought it was a little unusual that I couldn't recognize anyone and my surroundings looked different. I sat up and headed towards the restroom. When I came out I thought about checking on my brother. I walked over to his bed and saw another man was sleeping in it. I became upset with the person in my brother's bed and shouted at him "Hey! What are you doing in this bed? I need you to get out of this bed before my brother returns! Get up!" The guy opened his eyes confused looking up at me standing over him. He looked visibly ill and didn't seem to have the energy to engage me in a dispute. I insisted again that he get out of my brother's bed and threatened that I would call the nurses to remove him. Then a man in bed behind me interrupted and said "Sis. excuse Sis. Are you looking for the guy that was in that bed 2 days ago?" I responded "What do you mean two days ago? I left my brother here and went to get some rest. And I've returned to be with my brother but I found this guy in his bed."

He replied, "Sis, the person that was in that bed died two days ago, they've given his bed to someone else." I responded, "But how? I was just here with my brother earlier today." He again replied "No Sis, nobody has been over here for a couple of days now." I looked around and noticed different surroundings and many unfamiliar faces. It was in that stage that I began to accept the fact that my brother did perish while I was asleep. But, I still couldn't believe I've slept for a couple of days.

I walked outside, sat on a bench and stared at the sky. I was asking myself, "Why is this happening? How much more of this can I take? Now I am all alone." I began thinking about my life before ebola. I was remembering my family, my kids, our house and the community. I was stunned by how life has drastically changed for me. The memories and thoughts evoked a mixture of emotions. I cried, smiled, got angry and scared. After a few hours of deep thoughts I decided to return into the hospital building.

When I walked back into the hospital building I was approached by a familiar nurse. She stopped and stared at me in shock. She shouted "Hey everybody! Look at Angeline. She's walking around! She's doing well!" I was puzzled at her reason for the behavior. I asked her "What do you mean I am walking around?" She replied, "Are you serious?! You have been very ill laying in bed for a couple of days. You could barely open your mouth to take your medicine or even eat your food. We had to force feed you." This was strange to me because it felt like I've only slept for a few hours. I learned that my children's father had visited and brought me some goods while I was asleep.

I became aware about my condition, I realized that I was easily walking around without any help. Then it dawned on me, I was feeling better and recovering from the ebola virus. I felt happy and relieved. I looked around the hospital and noticed many people in worse condition. I saw people coughing, some vomiting and others crying out for help. A sight that still haunts me is that of a corpse sitting in a chair with her mouth opened and teeth exposed, she looked like a vampire.

As I kept walking through the hospital I noticed a person from my community, his name was Fody. Fody was the community ambulance driver that promised to transfer my father to the hospital but never showed up. I approached Fody because I wasn't going to miss the opportunity to express my disappointment of him abandoning my Father. I walked over to his bed and said, "Fody, is this you? Is this Fody the Ambulance driver that refused to help my father when he needed it the most?" Fody recognized me and turned his head to the opposite direction. I continued, "I guess we all ended up in the same place and infected by the same virus." He took a moment and then turned to look at me, "I am sorry. I was afraid and didn't want to catch the virus." I responded, "And how did that work out for you? We're both here fighting for our lifes at the Ebola hospital. I'm curious, how did you get infected by the virus?"

Fody stated he was transporting a young girl infected by the Ebola virus and she vomited on his foot. I noticed Fody's condition was pretty bad so I decided to pardon him and offered him my friendship. We briefly chatted about our community discussing other neighbors affected by the virus. I told Fody the location of my bed and suggested we stay in touch and fight this virus together.

The days went by and I could feel improvements to my health, my appetite and strength began to return. I was eating normal food and consistently taking the medicines that were provided to me. I noticed that every now and then the Doctor called a recovered patient's name and they were advised to return to their communities. I spoke to the Doctor and inquired about my desire to return to my house. The Doctor acknowledged my improvements and estimated I could be fully healed in a week. Three days later as I sat chatting with Fody, the Doctor approached me and said, "Guess what! Today is your day to return to your community!" I was elated.

As I collected my belongings, I was visited and congratulated by the nurses and a few friends I'd made during my stay at the Ebola Management Center. I then noticed my appearance and became concerned. I needed to fix my hair and put myself together before I returned home. My skin had turned darker than before, but I didn't care. I wanted the community and my family to see me in a fully recovered state.

V

I exited the hospital, walked onto the street's sidewalk and signaled a Taxi. The car stopped and as I opened the door to get in, a male passenger realized I was coming out of the Ebola Center. He immediately urged me to leave the Taxi stating, "Get out! I will not share a taxi with this Ebola woman!" I got into the Taxi and ignored the belligerent passenger.

I was feeling anxious when I arrived at the house. I was welcomed with support and happiness from my relatives and my children. They expressed their astonishment, they did not expect any of us would survive the Ebola virus. I delivered the sad news of my brother and sister at the hospital, we grieved their deaths together. I told them about Fody, the ambulance driver who was also at the hospital infected by the virus. The family gathered around and I narrated my Ebola survival story at the ELWA Center.

Even though I had survived and was discharged from the hospital, the illness' stigma still persisted. My family and neighbors kept an evident distance from me. My relatives wouldn't touch the dishes, pans and plates used by me and they refused to sit in any chair I've sat in. I also perceived similar treatment from the community members. Whenever I shopped at the grocery store, the clerk would refuse to take my money. But instead he would say "Keep your money and accept this item as a blessing." I grew tired of the ill treatment and decided to move to a new community far away from my old life, where no one knew my past. In March

2015 I received my official "EBOLA SURVIVOR CERTIFICATE OF DISCHARGE" which guaranteed I was no longer infectious nor a threat to the community.

I am deeply grateful to God for sparing my life even though I lost most of my family members. I can't explain how or why I survived and why my father, stepmother and siblings died. My only advice to everyone in the world is to take care of yourselves and stay mindful of these deadly viruses. We need to be mindful of the food we eat, wash our hands and protect ourselves. My name is Angeline Teah and this was my Ebola survival story.

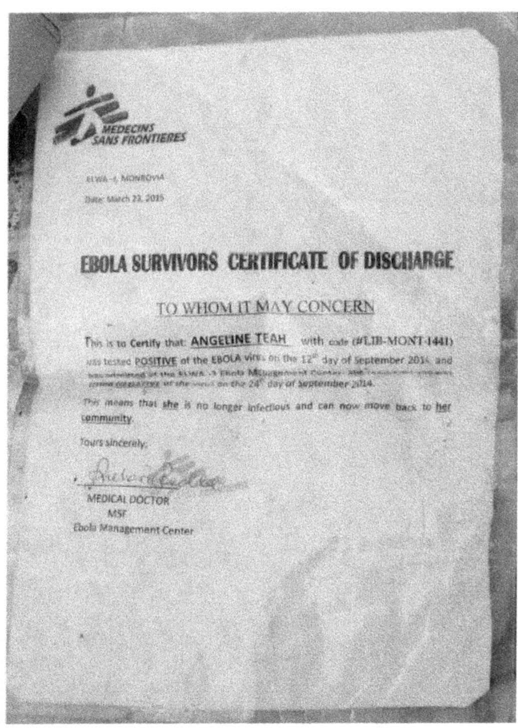

Ebola Survivors
Certificate of Discharge